MY JOURNAL

BALANCE YOUR BODY

BALANCE YOUR LIFE

Dr. Taub's 28-Day *Permanent* Weight Loss Plan

EDWARD A. TAUB, M.D.

k

KENSINGTON BOOKS
AND HEALTH VENTURES PARTNERS LLC

THIS KENSINGTON BOOK WAS CO-PUBLISHED BY:

Kensington Publishing Corp.
850 Third Avenue
New York, NY 10022

Health Ventures Partners LLC
c/o QVC, Inc.
Studio Park
West Chester, PA 19380

COPYRIGHT © 1999 BY EDWARD A. TAUB, M.D.

All rights reserved. No part of this book may be reproduced in any form or by any means without prior written consent of the Publisher, excepting brief quotes used in reviews.

Kensington and the K logo Reg. U.S. Pat. & TM Off.

ISBN 1-57566-437-2

First Printing: February 1999
10 9 8 7 6 5 4 3 2

Printed in the United States of America

YOUR 2-DAY PERSONAL
WELLNESS RETREAT

Please remember these next 2 days are about:

- Healthy Food
- Fresh Air
- Exercise
- Good Reading
- Soft Music
- Quiet Time For Meditation, Writing and Prayer

Please try to avoid:

- Television
- Telephone Calls
- Movies
- Newspapers
- Radio
- Unnecessary Interruptions

Some reminders

1. REMEMBER, THIS IS YOUR PERSONAL TIME!
2. NUTRITION: Be sure you have selected all your foods properly.
3. PHYSICAL ACTIVITY: Please follow the guide in the book.
4. JOURNAL: Take some time for writing at least twice each day.
5. BALANCE YOUR BODY, BALANCE YOUR LIFE: Be sure to have the book with you.

YOUR PERSONAL WELLNESS RETREAT SCHEDULE

Each day of your Personal Wellness Retreat requires about three or four hours of your time to accomplish essential and enjoyable tasks.

During the mornings, you'll need about one hour:

- 10–20 minutes for simple "wellness yoga" stretches
- 20 minutes for a "wellness walk"
- 20 minutes for meditation and journal writing

During the afternoon of each day, you'll need less than one hour:

- 20 minutes for a "wellness walk" in the afternoon (optional)
- 20 minutes for meditation and journal writing

Additionally, during the latter part of each day, you'll need between one and two hours:

- 1–2 hours for envisioning your future (Day One)
- 1–2 hours for doing a reality check (Day Two)

 TIME TO FOCUS ON YOU!

DAY ONE

CREATING YOUR VISION

When your mind is exceptionally clear, and you are feeling in a peak state (sometime during the latter part of the first day, after you've done your wellness yoga stretching, meditation and wellness walking), set aside at least an hour of time to answer the questions below as honestly and completely as possible.

First, take some time to review your answers to the Health Profile in Part Two of the book. This will give you many new insights and ideas. You will be building a *new path of least resistance* to the vision you are about to create, so be sure to come back to your journal at any time to make any additions. After you read each question below, close your eyes and ponder your answer, then write your answers in your journal on the following page. This will help keep your thoughts focused. Make sure that no one will disturb your concentration as you identify the following:

"Where I Want To Be One Year From Now"

- One year from today, how much do I want to weigh?
- After achieving this weight, what three characteristics most describe my life?
- What will I be doing for fun, and how much fun will I be having?
- What kind of exercise will I be doing?
- What will my body look like?
- What will my spouse or "special loved one" think of me?
- What will my children think of me?
- What will my health be like?
- What will my finances look like and where will I be in my career?
- How much will I respect myself?
- How much alcohol will I be drinking?
- How many cigarettes will I be smoking?
- Where will I be living?
- How loved will I feel?
- How loving will I be?

DAY ONE

Name: _____

Address: _____

Telephone: (   )   Date: /   /

LOCATION OF MY 2-DAY WELLNESS RETREAT:

_____
_____
_____

_____
_____
_____
_____
_____
_____
_____
_____
_____
_____
_____

DAY ONE

DAY ONE

DAY ONE

DAY ONE

 # DAY ONE

DAY ONE

DAY ONE

 # DAY ONE

DAY ONE

 # DAY ONE

DAY TWO

REALITY CHECK

The *Reality Check* may be an emotional jolt, and perhaps somewhat painful, but it is critical in progressing toward becoming leaner. It is meant to be a wake-up call.

During the second day of your Personal Wellness Retreat, take some time to once again review your Health Profile in Part Two of the book, then spend at least five mintues standing in front of a mirror with all or most of your clothes off. Treat what you see with honesty but kindness. Look especially at your face, arms, chest, abdomen, hips, thighs, buttocks and legs. Also look at your skin and hair. Notice your natural curves. After you are finished observing your body, write down your thoughts in your journal.

Now, write down your answers to the following questions as thoughtfully and completely as possible on the following page.

"Where I Am Right Now"

- How much do I weigh right now?
- What three characteristics most describe my life?
- What am I doing for fun, and how much fun am I having?
- What kind of exercises do I do?
- What kinds of physical pain am I experiencing?
- How sedentary ("couch potato") am I?
- What does my body look like?
- What does my spouse or "special loved one" think of me?
- What do my children think of me?
- What is my health like?
- What are my finances like and where am I in my career?
- How much do I respect myself?
- How much alcohol do I drink?
- How many cigarettes do I smoke?
- How stressed am I?
- How loved do I feel?
- How loving am I?

DAY TWO

DAY TWO

DAY TWO

DAY TWO

 # DAY TWO

DAY TWO

DAY TWO

DAY TWO

DAY TWO

DAY TWO

DAY TWO

FUTURE REALITY CHECK

Now imagine how you will be five years from now if you continue to live and eat as you currently do. Write down the answers to the following questions on the next page as honestly and completely as possible:

"This Describes Me Five Years From Now, If I Continue To Follow My Present Lifestyle And Eating Habits"

- How much will I weigh?
- What three characteristics will most describe my life?
- What will I be doing for fun, and how much fun will I be having?
- What kind of exercise will I be doing?
- What kinds of physical pain will I be experiencing?
- How sedentary will I be?
- What will my body look like?
- What will my spouse or "special loved one" think of me?
- What will my children think of me?
- What will my health be like?
- What will my finances look like and where will I be in my career?
- How much will I respect myself?
- How much alcohol will I be drinking?
- How many cigarettes will I be smoking?
- Where will I be living?
- How stressed will I be?
- How loved will I be?
- How loving will I be?

FUTURE REALITY CHECK

FUTURE REALITY CHECK

FUTURE REALITY CHECK

FUTURE REALITY CHECK

FUTURE REALITY CHECK

YOUR 28-DAY
PERMANENT
WEIGHT LOSS PLAN

BE SURE YOU HAVE YOUR COPY OF
BALANCE YOUR BODY, BALANCE YOUR LIFE
WITH YOU SO YOU CAN REFERENCE
THE FOLLOWING:

- Every day, write down at least one thing you are proud of for that day—***EMPHASIZE THE POSITIVE!***

- Remember, it is important to stay among the top five steps of the **FOOD ENERGY LADDER** for most of the next 28 days.

- Every day, be sure to do your *wellness yoga stretching* and your *wellness walking*.

- Every day, before and after you finish your *mental relaxation exercises*, write down how you are feeling.

- Remember, you have strength!

THE FOOD ENERGY LADDER

1	FRUITS	1
2	VEGETABLES	2
3	PASTA • RICE • POTATOES	3
4	WHOLE GRAIN BREADS • CEREALS	4
5	NUTS • AVOCADOS • OLIVE OIL	5
6	FISH	6
7	POULTRY	7
8	BEEF • PORK • LAMB • VEAL	8
9	LOW-FAT DAIRY PRODUCTS	9
10	REGULAR DAIRY PRODUCTS	10
11	EGGS	11
12	CANDY • SWEETS	12

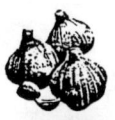

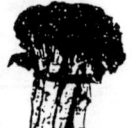

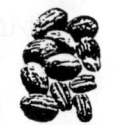

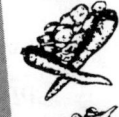

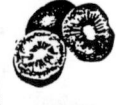

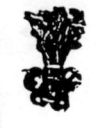

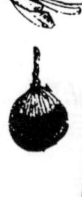

"Everything in moderation, including moderation."

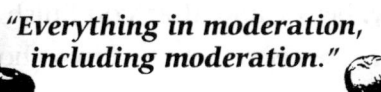

DAY 1

If you want your dreams to come true, don't sleep, act!

—YIDDISH PROVERB

DAY 2

Our greatest glory is not in never falling, but in rising every time we fall.

—CONFUCIUS

DAY 3

The world cares very little about what a man or woman knows; it is what a man or woman is able to do that counts.

—BOOKER T. WASHINGTON

DAY 4

It's okay to make mistakes. Mistakes are our teachers—they help us to learn.

—JOHN BRADSHAW

DAY 5

Look at a day when you are supremely satisfied at the end. It's not a day when you lounge around doing nothing, it's when you've had everything to do, and you've done it.

—MARGARET THATCHER

DAY 6

The only place where your dream becomes impossible is in your own thinking.

—ROBERT H. SCHULLER

DAY 7

There is hunger for ordinary bread but there is also hunger for love, for kindness and for thoughtfulness. This is the great poverty that makes people suffer so much.

—MOTHER TERESA

DAY 8

If opportunity doesn't knock, build a door.
—MILTON BERLE

DAY 9

Look after yourself every day and put forth your best effort to love yourself enough to do what's best.

—OPRAH WINFREY

DAY 10

You must do the very thing you think you cannot do.

—ELEANOR ROOSEVELT

DAY 11

We all have ability. The difference is how we use it.

—STEVIE WONDER

DAY 12

They can conquer who believe they can. He has not learned the first lesson of life who does not every day surmount a fear.

—RALPH WALDO EMERSON

DAY 13

We can do anything *we* want if we stick to it long enough.

—HELEN KELLER

DAY 14

If I'd known I was gonna live this long, I'd have taken better care of myself.

—EUBIE BLAKE AT AGE 100

❧ DAY 15

Dining is, after all, a spiritual experience.
—NICOS KAZANTAKIS

DAY 16

Strength does not come from physical capacity. It comes from an indomitable will.

—MAHATMA GANDHI

DAY 17

When you win . . . you won't remember the pain.
—JOE NAMATH

DAY 18

The ultimate measure of a man is not where he stands in moments of comfort and convenience, but where he stands in times of challenge.

—MARTIN LUTHER KING

DAY 19

We write our own destiny. We become what we do.

—MADAME CHIANG KAI-SHEK

DAY 20

Never wait for trouble. Be prepared for it.
—CHUCK YAEGER

DAY 21

The doctor of the future will give no medicine, but will interest his patients in the care of the human frame, in diet, and in the cause of disease.

—THOMAS EDISON

DAY 22

Every blade of grass has its Angel that bends over it and whispers, *"Grow . . . Grow."*

—THE TALMUD

DAY 23

Resolve, and you are free!
—HENRY WADSWORTH LONGFELLOW

DAY 24

Never let the fear of striking out get in your way.
—BABE RUTH

DAY 25

The journey of a thousand miles begins with one step.

—LAO-TSZE

DAY 26

The whole of science is nothing more than a refinement of everyday thinking.

—ALBERT EINSTEIN

DAY 27

Everyone's life is a fairy tale written by God's fingers.
—HANS CHRISTIAN ANDERSON

DAY 28

Start the day with love. Fill the day with love. End the day with love.

—SATHYA SAIBABA